HEALTH *without* WEALTH

How to Eat Healthy and Save Money

NADINE ALLENIE

TABLE OF CONTENTS

INTRODUCTION

I want to thank you for choosing this book, '*Health without Wealth: How to Eat Healthy and Save Money.*'

Have you been putting off eating healthy because you think healthy food doesn't fit your budget? Do you believe that eating healthy would mean eating a lot of junk food and devoiding yourself of nutrition?

Over the years, the mainstream media has made us believe that the only way to eat healthy is to buy expensive and exotic looking food items that apparently are full of nutrition as compared to the cheaper ingredients. I get it. I have been there too! There was a time where I thought eating caviar, steak or other such overpriced foods could be my ticket to leading a healthy life. And for about six months, I bought the most expensive foods around because I was trying to build some muscle.

Of course, within a short period of time, I realized that it was also drilling a big hole in my pocket and that it couldn't go on like this. It finally dawned upon me that I could choose not to spend ridiculous amounts of money on food and still eat healthy.

This book offers some valuable insights on how you can eat healthy while on a budget. I wanted to create a guide that educates my readers about the nutrition present in some of the simplest and cheapest food available. You will also learn some tips as to how you can save some more money by simply changing your habits.

Making a grocery list, meal planning or buying on sale are some of easiest ways of ensuring that you don't buy on an impulse.

If you follow the tips given in this book, you will never find yourself in an awkward position where you have to choose between your budget and eating healthy. Happy reading!!

CHAPTER ONE

Debunking Myths about Eating Healthy

Healthy equals expensive

Most people think that eating healthy means destroying their budgets, and that's false. There are many ways to ensure that you save some money and still eat healthy. Being a savvy shopper, taking into account some meal planning tactics, learning to cook at home or packing your lunches can certainly help you stay within your budget. You can find more such tips in the following chapter about budget eating.

Local marketplace doesn't sell healthy food

Let me ask you this. How long has it been since you last visited the local marketplace? I am guessing most of you don't even know where it is. We have got into the habit of ordering food from the supermarket without looking around for alternatives that can actually save you some money. In fact, if you do take out the time to look around, you will find that the local marketplace is full of items that can help you eat healthier. Spend some time in aisles looking for organic meats, frozen produce and wholegrain products.

Healthy cooking takes too much time

Cooking healthy doesn't mean that you spend an entire day in the kitchen. Simple cooking methods such as steaming or sautéing could take only a few minutes. Chicken can be baked within 25 minutes, rice can be cooked under 20 minutes in a rice cooker and a vegetable salad can be prepared in merely 10 minutes. You can also use a crockpot, which allows you to dump all the ingredients in it and relax while the food is cooking away.

Frozen fruit and veggies are not healthy

When you freeze fruit and veggies, it locks in their flavors and nutrients. In fact, frozen produce is ideal for people who are looking to adopt better eating habits. Even some of the top most chefs rely on frozen produce, as they are more wholesome and flavorful as compared to canned veggies.

You must eat meat every single day

No, you don't have to! Not every single meal you eat should consist of meat in order for it to be healthy. If you think meat is the only way you can have a filling meal, consider replacing it with red beans, black beans and white navy beans and it will turn out just as satiating and tasty. There are several alternatives when it comes to replacing the protein present in meats. Nuts, tofu or lentils along with a variety of other veggies contain plenty of protein.

All fats are bad

Low-fat meals are never considered as being tempting. Regardless of how many negative things you have heard about fats, you should know that not all fats are bad. And these fats don't necessarily have to come from expensive foods. You can include nuts, beans or sunflower seeds to your diet to fulfill your fat requirements.

CHAPTER TWO

Ways to Eat on a Budget

Now that we have debunked some of the most popular myths about healthy eating let's see how can eat healthy on a budget.

Make a grocery list and Stick to it

Take some time out to make a grocery list and stick to it. It's easy to get tempted to buy things that are not on the list when you head out to a grocery store. Once you get sidetracked, you may end up making expensive as well as irrelevant purchases. As a rule, each time you hit the grocery store, start shopping from the perimeter of the store. This is where the most inexpensive as well as healthy foods are kept. If you notice, it's the middle of the store where the most unhealthy and most processed food items are stacked up. Avoid getting lost in these aisles by checking your list every few minutes. Alternatively, you can also use grocery apps that can help you make the right purchases.

Cook at home

Have a good look at your monthly expenses – chances are that most of you spend your money on eating out. I get it. It's fun to visit a restaurant and eat your favorite foods without having to put in any effort. For some of you, it's the ambiance that makes you want to hit different restaurants and it's completely okay, but how much is too much? If it's destroying your budget and making you stress over your finances, then you need to reconsider your choices. If you do the math, you can feed a family of four for an equal amount of money that you end up paying for two people in a restaurant. Think about it. Wouldn't that save you unnecessary expenditure? Make it a habit to cook simple food that is nutritious and easy to make. If you can't find the time to cook every day, plan your meals, cook them in batches and store them in airtight containers in the refrigerator for future use. When you start to work closely with food, you will know exactly why a certain food is beneficial for health and how you can find a cheaper version of it without compromising on the quality.

Do not shop when you are hungry

Don't shop when you are ravenously hungry as that will distract you from your grocery list and make you impulsive. Most people don't plan their weekly shopping and only hit the grocery store when they have run out of groceries at home. You need to organize your schedule such a manner that you have enough ingredients in your kitchen for an entire week. Personally, I prefer loading up my kitchen with food every 3 weeks. Doing this not only saves me time, but also saves me from the hassle of having to shop every week. That being said, if you absolutely have to shop when you are hungry, then try to grab some fruit, a cup of yogurt or a smoothie before you hit the store. This will help prevent you from buying out of impulse when you are out shopping.

Buy whole foods

I know a lot of people who spend extravagant amounts of money buying bottled juices, which are being marketed as organic or healthy. Why not buy some fresh fruit instead? Do you know that it's actually much healthier to eat whole fruit rather than juicing them? The same goes with whole foods. For instance, buying blocked cheese instead of shredded cheese or buying canned beans instead of refried beans is not only healthier, but cheaper on your pocket too. Whole grains such as oats or brown rice are inexpensive and offer you're a lot of nutrition per serving as compared to most processed cereals. Buying them in larger quantities can also get you more discounts.

Buy generic brands

There are several stores that offer generic brands for almost any product. And if you think that generic means low quality, think again! Every food manufacturer is required to follow certain standards when it comes to food. They are lawfully responsible to provide safe food to the customers. So, there's no question of the food quality being compromised. These generic brands actually sell the same quality as several national brands, but are inexpensive. However, you need to go through the list of the ingredients printed at the back of every packet to ensure that the product you are buying contains quality ingredients. As long as you do your research before you head out to buy food items from these generic brands, you won't go far wrong.

Cut junk from your diet

No, this isn't only good for your weight loss, but it's great for your finances too. You may be surprised to find out how much you are spending for colas, fries, cookies and processed foods. Besides the fact that none of these food items offer any nutrition and only add to your daily calorific limit, they are also very expensive. Now, it may seem difficult to give up on all processed food if you have been a processed food junkie for years. Realistically speaking, you can start by cutting down on one junk item that you would normally eat every week, and then gradually move to on eliminating the rest of them. Remember that it's a slow process and if you try to give up on all the junk in a day, the cravings may actually come back with a vengeance, and you may end up eating more junk and spending more money. Once you get into the habit of skipping unhealthy or processed food items, you can concentrate on buying quality foods that are healthier as well as cheaper.

Watch out for sales

Be on the lookout for monthly sales at the nearby grocery store. If your favorite products or staples are on sale, you should buy them in bulk to save some money. However, be careful about your purchase during the sale – avoid buying things you don't need. If you are completely sure that the items put up on sale are useful then you might as well stock them up to save bit of money. Another thing to remember is to make sure that the products you are buying won't expire too soon and are long-lasting. It doesn't make sense to buy something just because it is cheaper, only to find out later that it's close to its expiration date.

Look for cheaper cuts of meat

If you are a meat lover, you might end up spending extra money as meat and fish can be quite expensive. However, you can also buy cheaper cuts of meat that cost way less than the normal meat. You can use them in soups, sandwiches, burritos, and stews and stir-fries. It can also help to buy a large portion of meat and then store it in the refrigerator for the entire week. You can also clean the meat, and cut it in chunks so they can easily fit in the boxes. The same applies to fish.

Buy produce that is in season

Local produce that is in season is generally sold at cheaper rates. This type of produce is also rich in nutrients and flavor. When you buy food that is canned and not in season, you make yourself vulnerable to allergies. Produce that is not in season is transported halfway across the globe so that it can get to your store, and by the time it reaches you, it loses its nutritional value and also cost you more. You can also buy produce by the bag, which will cost you much less than buying by the piece. If you happen to buy more than what you need, you can simply wrap the ingredients and freeze them for a couple of weeks until further use.

Purchase frozen veggies and fruit

Certain fruit and vegetables are generally in season only some months every year and can sometimes be extremely expensive. Here's a simple solution – you can buy quick-frozen produce, which is just as nutritious and doesn't cost you much. Such produce is available all through the year and is usually sold in large bags. Frozen produce is also known to enhance the flavor of the dish. You can use it while making smoothies, baking, or as a topping for your morning cereal. Moreover, it also allows you to take out only as much as you require while cooking so the rest can be stored back in the freezer until you are ready to use it again. This saves you a lot of wastage.

Grow your own produce

Now this may seem unrealistic to some of you, but trust me, it's not as difficult or as time consuming as you think. Think about it - what can be more satisfying than treating yourself to delicious meals made out of your own produce? If you didn't know this already, seeds are very inexpensive and can be bought easily from stores or online. If you put in some time every day, combined with a little bit of effort, you will be able to grow your own tomatoes, chilies, onions, coriander, herbs and many such delicious crops. When you have a constant supply of fresh produce at home, you will not only eat healthy, but also saves you money that you generally spend in the stores. Homegrown produce is also tastier and more nutritious than the store-brought produce. Also, you can be sure that the produce is picked when it's at its peak of ripeness.

Pack your lunch

If you spend most of your time in the office, chances are that you eat at least two of your meals at your workplace. Do you pack your lunch or eat out every day? Eating out can get expensive if done regularly. Packing your lunch, on the other hand, allows you to dig into some healthy meals at lower costs. If you have got into the habit of cooking your own meals, packing your meals and carrying them to your workplace will only make your life easier. However, if you don't want to learn how to cook, you can pack yourself some fruit, nuts or raw veggies (carrots and cucumbers) to take to the office. Now this does require some planning, but it will be worth your effort.

Appreciate inexpensive foods

How many times do we take the inexpensive foods for granted? Carrots, cucumbers, certain fruit, whole grains and even eggs are not only inexpensive, but they also provide the same nutrition that some of the most expensive foods have to offer. Start to appreciate these foods and make the best use of them. Instead of buying yourself exotic juices and cheeses, gorge on these simple yet nutritious and tastier foods to save some money. Incorporating these foods in your daily diet might need some time, but it will help you eat well without spending a fortune on expensive food items.

Buy from online retailers

Do you know that there are several online retailers who sell healthy foods at 50% discount? You can easily register yourself online and get access to daily deals and discounts. What's more, if you download their app, these retailers will even deliver the products to your door, sometimes, even free of cost. For starters, you can try using thrive retailer which focuses on selling unprocessed and healthy foods. They also offer you different payment options, sometimes even credit for your purchases.

CHAPTER THREE

Seven-day Muscle Building Diet Plan

You really don't have to worry about having enough money to buy yourself nutritious foods if your goal is to build muscle. We are recommending a seven day diet plan which promises to deliver all your carbohydrate and protein needs you require to fuel yourself through the training. Instead of spending a fortune on exotic looking veggies or pricey slabs of chicken breasts, we are giving you an option of pork steaks, turkey burgers and chicken thighs which contain the same nutrition, but at a cheaper price.

Buy in Bulk

There are several food delivery companies that offer huge discounts for big orders. Ordering food from such companies will not only save you money, but also save you the hassle of having to go the grocery store often. Instead of simply grabbing unhealthy ingredients on your way back home, you can order nutritious foods like nut butters or chicken thighs from these companies. Another thing you can do is to order the food list on a weekend so you can whip up a delicious meal right away whenever you want to.

Batch cook Sundays

Once you get the ingredients delivered, you can start organizing your meals. If you are always on a busy schedule, chances are that you don't get enough time to spend in the kitchen. Rather than cooking every day, you can set aside some time every Sunday to batch cook your meals. Soups, broths, stews, casseroles, sandwiches or even curries can be stored in air-tight containers in the refrigerator, saving you loads of kitchen labor after a long day at work. Now the hardest part about this trick is that you will have to exercise some amount of self-control to not eat everything at once. Nevertheless, it's still easier than having to spend hours in the kitchen without leaving you with any "me time."

Pick frozen over fresh

Since fresh ingredients have a shorter shelf life, they need to be used up quickly, and this can mean more hassle. Instead, stock your fridge with loads of frozen veggies and fruit. Similarly, you can store meats, tuna and even beans inside your freezer. Apart from offering convenience, the freezing method also preserves the flavor and the nutritional value of the ingredients, plus frozen food is also cheaper. You can take them out just a little before breakfast, lunch or dinner and use a crockpot or a microwave to cook them.

Monday

Breakfast: Poached eggs on spinach

Lunch: **whole-wheat flatbread with some frozen tuna, onion and tomato**

Snack: Greek yogurt with berries and nuts

Dinner: **Sweet potato, roasted cauliflower and steamed salmon**

Tuesday

Breakfast: rolled oats porridge with milk and bananas

Lunch: fried brown rice with veggies

Snack: fried peanuts

Dinner: Grilled pork steak in homemade tomato sauce

Wednesday

Breakfast: homemade peanut butter and egg whites

Lunch: carrot salad and mackerel with tomato

Snack: a glass of milk

Dinner: brown rice with kidney beans in tomato sauce

Thursday

Breakfast: 3 scrambled eggs with sausages

Lunch: leftover chili with sweet potato

Snack: peanut butter and brown bread

Dinner: garlic roasted chicken thighs

Friday

Breakfast: leftover chicken and mushroom omelet

Lunch: salmon and cottage cheese with brown rice

Snack: carrot sticks with hummus

Dinner: garlic roasted broccoli or cauliflower along with steak

Saturday

Breakfast: porridge with bananas, honey and almonds

Lunch: brown rice pilaf with green peas

Snack: pitta bread and cottage cheese

Dinner: green beans and cauliflower mash with prawn rice

Sunday

Breakfast: egg frittata, roasted broccoli and sausages

Lunch: turkey sandwiches (brown bread)

Snack: apples

Dinner: crockpot lamb stew with roasted sweet potato and peas

CHAPTER FOUR

Top Ten Cheap yet Healthy Foods

Brown rice

Brown rice costs only 10 cents per one-fourth cup serving and is much better for your health as compared to white rice. Here are some of the reasons why:

In order to make white rice, the first few layers of the rice grain are removed, resulting into a polished grain of rice which has lower nutritional value left. But brown rice is actually a wholegrain unlike the polished white rice. Even while processing the brown rice, only the hull is removed while the nutrition remains intact. Also, brown rice contains much more fiber and contains valuable minerals such as zinc and magnesium.

Beans

Beans are known to be extremely heart healthy and, not just that, but they are also a powerhouse food. Beans are full of protein and fiber along with healthy dietary fat. The low glycemic index of beans makes them release energy in your bloodstream, making you feel full and more satisfied. Since beans can be bought in bulk and dry, they are also very economical. There are several beans to choose from – pinto beans, black beans, red beans, garbanzo beans and much more. You can buy dry beans in cans and they won't cost you more than 50 cents per serving on an average.

Eggs

Eggs have received a lot of flak in the past few years, especially the egg yolk. Contrary to the popular belief, egg yolks don't contain a ton of cholesterol. In fact, many doctors today recommend eating one or two whole eggs to prevent stroke and heart disease. Eggs are also loaded with protein. One egg can offer as much as 11 percent of your per day protein intake. Eggs are also good for your skin, hair and overall diet. As per a particular study, people who consume eggs for breakfast every day are capable of losing twice as much weight as the ones who ate bagels –in spite of consuming the same amount of calories. Eggs can be bought for as low as $1.50 a dozen from any local grocery store.

Sweet potatoes

A lot of us eat sweet potatoes only during Thanksgiving or winter. However, they can be a great addition to a variety of dishes in your daily diet too. The best part is that sweet potatoes can be bought for just about a couple of bucks and are very satiating. They are also highly nutritious – sweet potatoes contain lot of fiber, calcium, Vitamin A and C and potassium. Sweet potatoes can also give you great skin, as they are loaded with antioxidants. Most dieters include sweet potatoes in their diets as they contain only 95 calories per serving.

Canned Tuna

Fish is great for your heart as well as the brain, but most people cannot afford restaurant-quality cuts. However, canned tuna that contains only 62 calories per serving can offer you the same amount of nutrients at a lower cost. Tuna contains a lot of vitamins and minerals and is also rich in omega-3 fatty acids. These acids can prevent you from developing cholesterol issues and lower your risk of heart disease or stroke by maintaining your blood pressure levels.

Bananas

Is there anything cooler than a banana? Bananas are completely portable and are loaded with nutrients and fiber. You can buy a single banana for as low as 40 cents. Banana is one of the cheapest foods as it is always available 12 months a year. They are also a great source of potassium; so if you are planning to run a marathon, just eat one or two bananas before the run to sustain your energy levels. Athletes love bananas because they contain vital potassium, which is essential to maintain energy. Bananas are also known to lower your risk of developing ulcers and constipation and also help protect your kidneys.

Whole-wheat Pasta

How about eating whole-wheat pasta instead of store-bought burgers? It is tastier, filling and nutritious as compared to any other junk or processed food. Whole-wheat pasta contains three times more fiber than regular pasta and is known to lower your risk for diabetes and heart disease. It is also very satiating, which means you will end up consuming less calories – resulting in weight loss. A typical box of whole-wheat pasta will cost you less than $2 and offers you an average of $28 per serving. Not bad eh?

Store-bought marinara sauce can be quite inexpensive as well, and you can simply pair it with your pasta for a delicious meal. You can also add whole-wheat pasta to your salads or sandwiches or dress it up with some boiled eggs and tuna with some vinegar.

Canned tomatoes

As per studies, when you cook certain foods, it allows the body to absorb the nutrients faster. One such food is the tomato. When cooked, tomatoes make it easier for the body to absorb a powerful antioxidant known as lycopene. If you combine the lycopene with a bit of fat, the absorption can happen even faster and better. Canned tomatoes can be very cost-effective meal starters. A single can of tomatoes can be bought for just about a dollar or even less when they are on sale.

Flank Steak

Here's some good news for meat lovers. You don't have to eliminate red meat from your diet completely in order to stay fit. All you need to do is pick the right cuts. Lean beef contains less saturated fat as compared to a regular cut and is much more economically priced. Flank steaks also contain a healthy amount of iron, protein, vitamins and zinc. Leaner cuts of beef are softer in texture and more delicious than the regular beef. More chefs recommend marinating the flank steaks overnight to reap the maximum flavor. These lean steaks can end up tasting even tastier than an expensive fillet.

Cottage cheese

A 16 oz. can of cottage cheese will cost you just about $2 and would be a great addition to your daily diet. Cottage cheese is also known to be a rich source of protein – half cup of cottage cheese contains as much as 14 grams of protein. It is also helpful to control your appetite while you are trying to lose some weight. Cottage cheese consists of a variety of nutrients including phosphorous and calcium, which are significant for bone health. It can also be enjoyed as a tasty snack – simply marinate it in some yogurt and mint for 20 minutes and stir fry the chunks in a pan until they are golden brown from all sides. Cottage cheese tastes even more flavorful when added to salads along with fruit.

CONCLUSION

I wish to thank all my readers for purchasing this book.

I bet you didn't think eating on a budget was that easy. Food doesn't need to be complicated, or bad, or expensive. Buying low-cost foods doesn't always mean that you will be giving up on its benefits.

I remember how my granny would prepare the tastiest and most nutritious meals out of simple foods such as buckwheat oats, millet, fruit and veggies without overspending. Can't we do the same? You can certainly enjoy eating out and allow yourself to gorge on expensive meals whenever you want to, but it doesn't have to be a regular feature of your lifestyle.

I hope this book was worth every penny you spend on this book. If you liked the tips given in the book, don't hesitate to pass them on to your friends and family members and don't forget to write a review for the book.

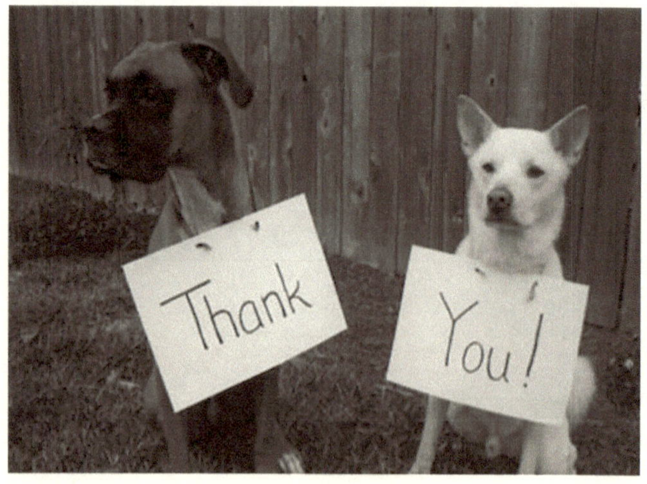

Finally, if you enjoyed this book then I'd like to ask you for a favor. Will you be kind enough to leave a review for this book on Amazon? It would be greatly appreciated!

Click here to leave a review for this book on Amazon!
Thank you and good luck!

REFERENCE:

https://recipes.howstuffworks.com/menus/10-healthy-cheap-foods10.htm

https://www.healthline.com/nutrition/19-ways-to-eat-healthy-on-a-budget#section3

http://www.coachmag.co.uk/nutrition/4042/try-this-7-day-muscle-building-diet-plan-it-s-super-cheap